NEW WEIGHT WATCHERS F]

Table of Contents

Chapter 1 : Breakfast
Chapter 2 : Vegetarian And Vegan Recipes
Chapter 3 : Chicken And Poultry Recipes
Chapter 4 : Fish And Seafood Recipes
Chapter 5 : Beef And Pork Recipes
Chapter 6 : Dessert

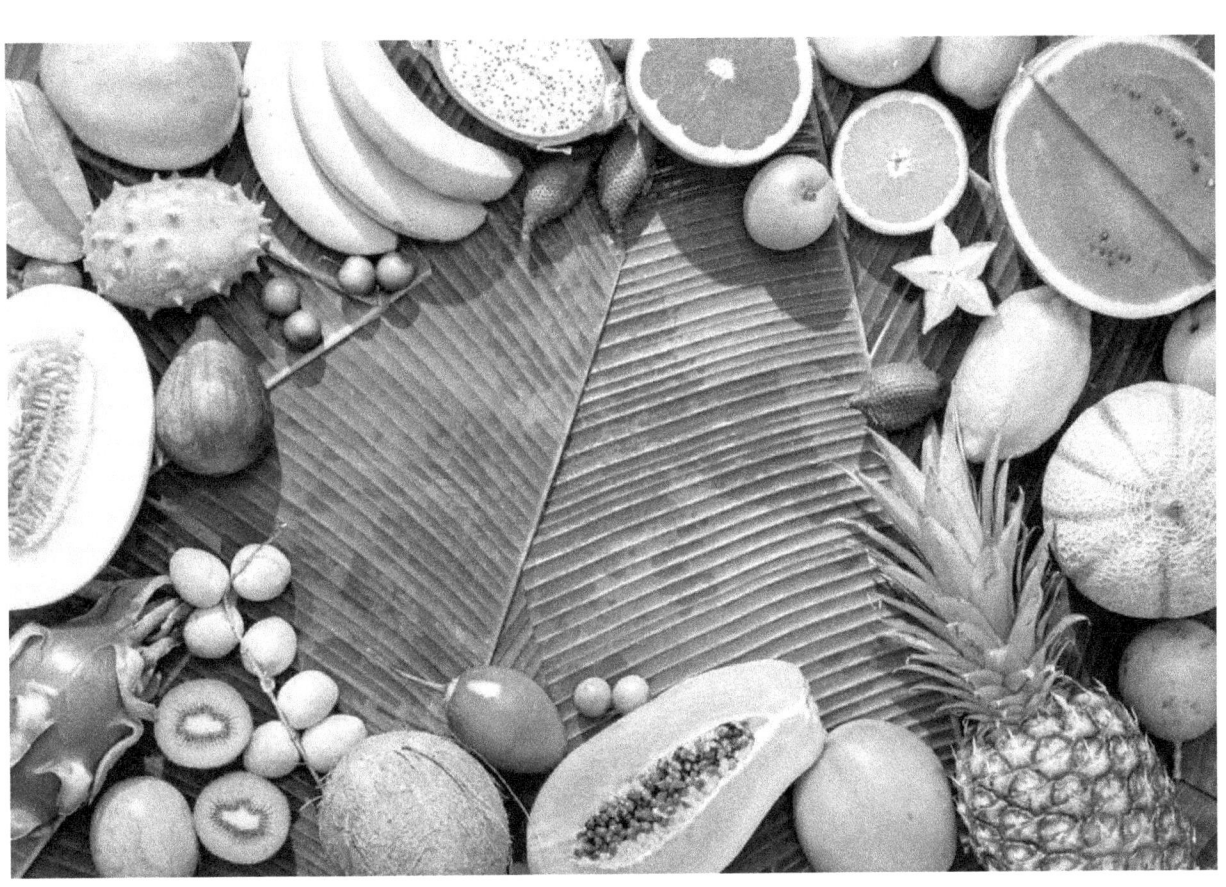

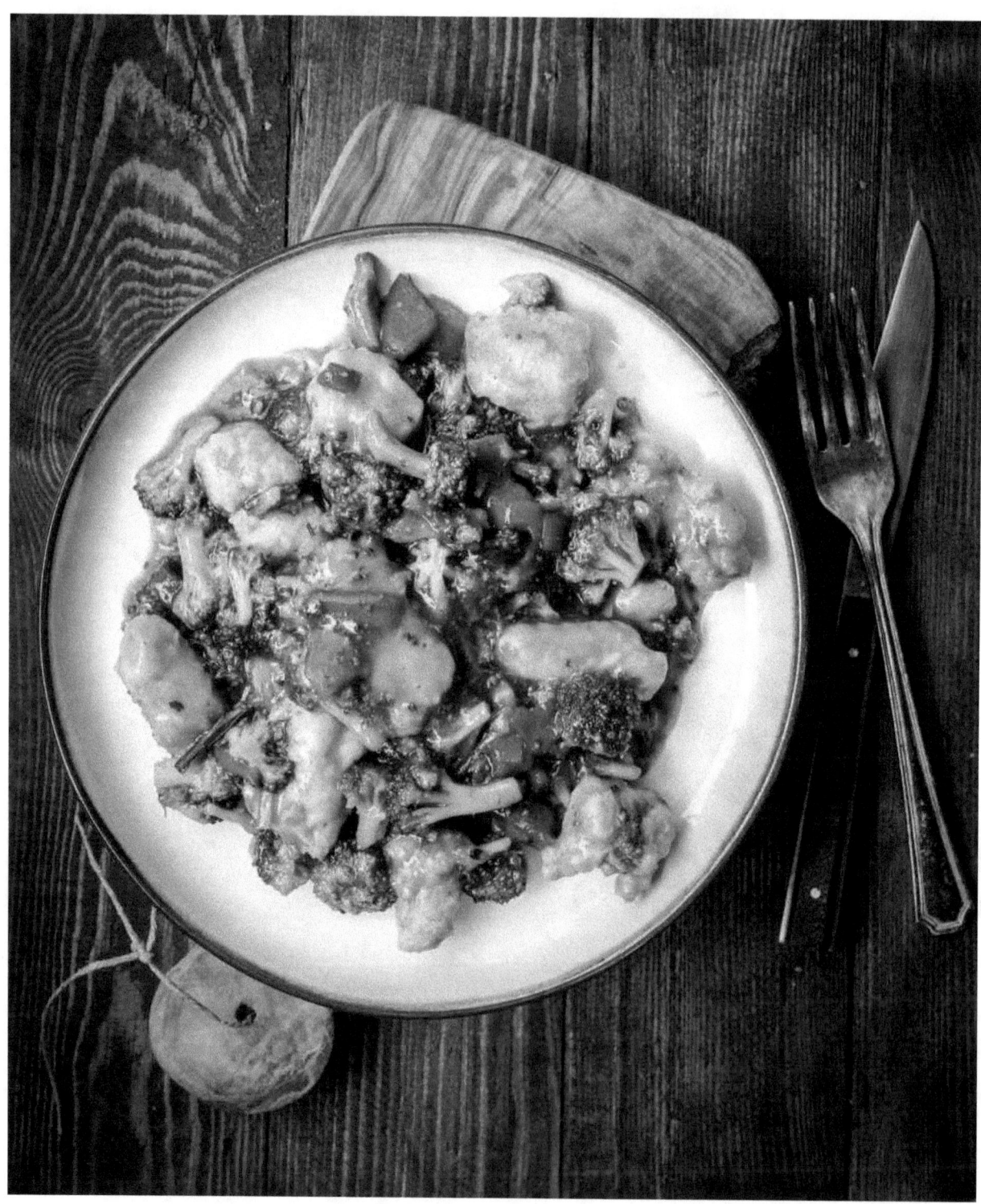

Copyright 2021 - All rights reserved.

All rights reserved. No part of this publication may be reproduced, distributed, or transmitted in any form or by any means, including photocopying, recording, or other electronic or mechanical methods, without the prior written permission of the publisher.

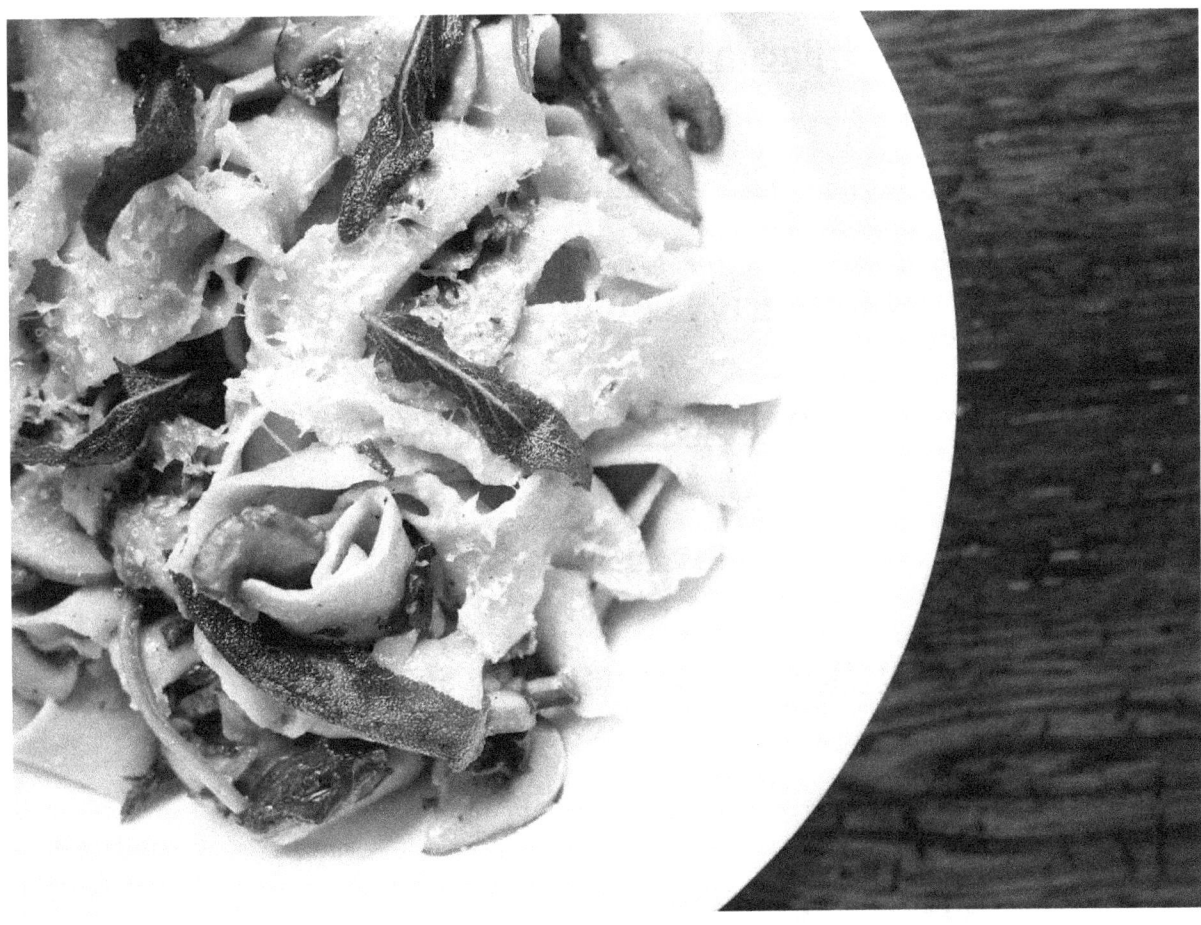

CONTENTS

Chapter 1: Breakfast

Lovely Pineapple Juice

Bacon And Cheese Quiche

Broccoli Egg Muffins

Delicious Almond Pancake

Homely Chicken Omelet

Simple Almond Cereal

Delicious Almond Berry Smoothie

Simple 3 Ingredient Pancake

Chapter 2: Vegetarian And Vegan Recipes

Melon And Watercress Salad

Beet And Mushroom Meal

Fresh Heirloom Carrot

Original Avocado Salad

Chapter 3: Chicken And Poultry Recipes

Hearty Balsamic Chicken

Epic Mango Chicken

Thick Broccoli And Cream Soup

Roasted Tomato Soup

Creative Green Soup

Turkey Green Bean Soup

Mesmerizing Orange Baked Chicken *

Cool Sheet-Pan Chicken Asparagus

Chapter 4: Fish And Seafood Recipes

Awesome Dijon Fish

Juicy Shrimp Scampi

Creamed Halibut

Classic Crab Cakes

Baked Garlic And Lemon Mahi Mahi

Lovely Mediterranean Fish

The Pan-Grilled Fish Steaks

Classic Meddieternean Fish

Simple Baked Mahi Mahi

Chapter 5: Beef And Pork Recipes

Caramelized Pork Chops And Onion

Mustard Lamb Cutlets

Beef Broccoli Dinner

Roast Taco Wraps

Grilled Spiced Chops

Beef Stuffed Zucchini

Subtle Herbed Beef Roast

Purely Spanish Pork Cutlets And Onion

Chapter 6: Dessert

Fine Baked Apple

Healthy Bean Balls

Cool Carrot Balls

Applesauce Bean Brownies

Pumpkin Cake Muffins

Fried Up Sliced Apples

Fluffy Almond Pancakes

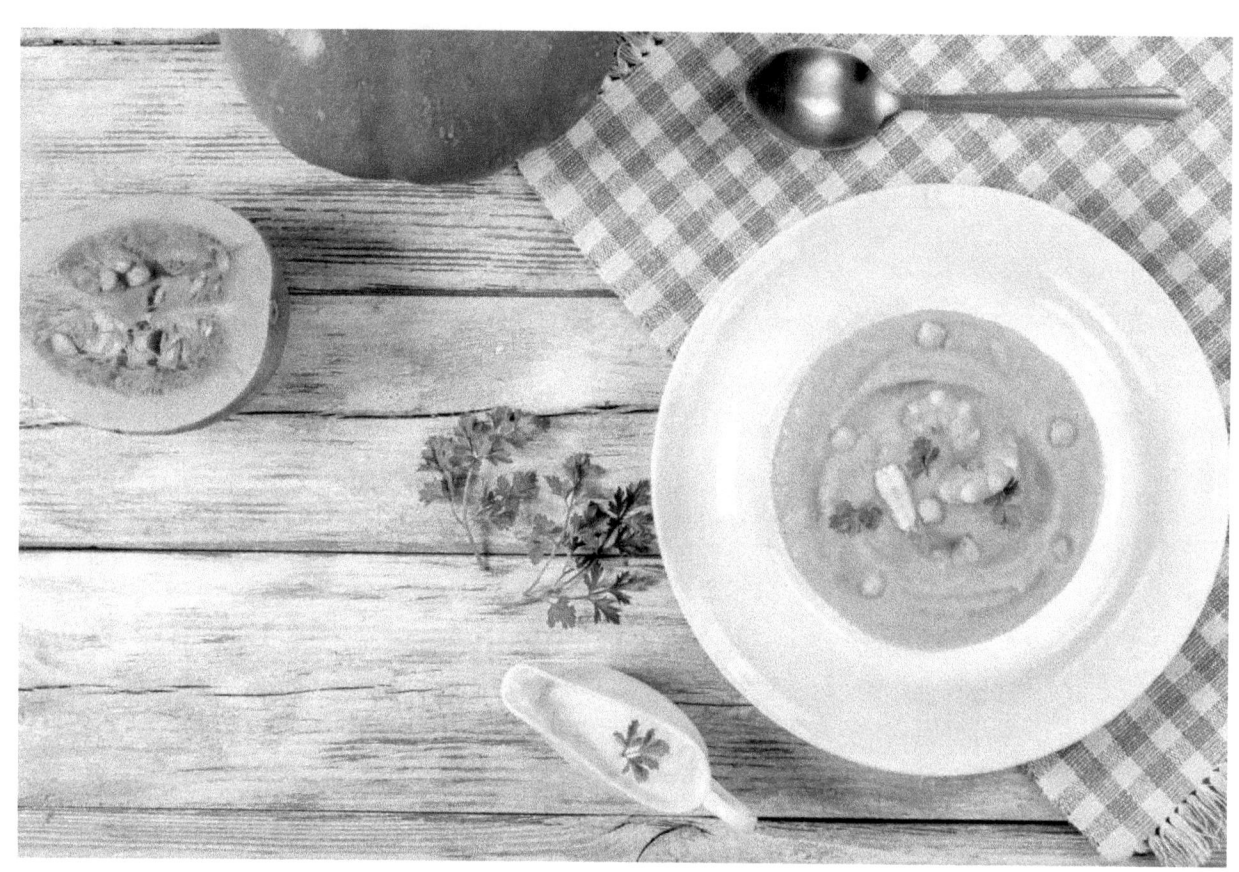

Chapter 1: Breakfast

Lovely Pineapple Juice

Prep Time: 10 minutes

Cooking Time: Nil

Number of Servings: 4

Ingredients:

- 4 cups of fresh pineapple, chopped
- 1 pinch of salt
- 1 and a ½ cup of water

Method:

1. Add the listed ingredients to your blender and blend well until you have a smoothie-like texture
2. Chill and serve
3. Enjoy!

Nutritional Values (Per Serving)

- Calories: 82
- Fat: 0.2 g
- Saturated Fat: 0 g
- Carbohydrates: 21 g
- Fiber: 0 g
- Sodium: 67 mg
- Protein: 21 g

Bacon And Chees Quiche

Prep Time: 10 minutes

Cooking Time: 30 minutes

Number of Servings: 4

SmartPoints: 4

Ingredients:

- 3 and a ½ ounce of raw Broccoli cut up into small florets
- 4 sprays of Calorie controlled cooking spray
- 3 rasher bacon medallions, raw and roughly chopped up
- 2 medium spring onions trimmed and sliced
- 2 and a ½ ounce of Reduce Fat Grated Cheese
- 2 medium raw whole eggs
- ½ a cup of skimmed milk
- 3 and a ½ ounce of low soft cheese

Method:

1. Preheat your oven to 356 degrees Fahrenheit
2. Cook broccoli in a pan of boiling water over medium heat and cook for 4 minutes
3. Drain and spread out layers in kitchen paper and allow them to dry
4. Take a nonstick frying pan and place it over medium heat
5. Grease with cooking spray and add bacon and spring onions, cook for 4:5 minutes
6. Take a 7 inch shallow round cake and grease with cooking spray
7. Spread broccoli and bacon mix over the base and scatter cheese
8. Season with black pepper
9. Beat the eggs, milk, soft cheese together
10. Pour into the tin and bake for 25 minutes
11. Enjoy!

Nutritional Values (Per Serving)

- Calories: 365
- Fat: 24 g
- Saturated Fat: 3 g

- Carbohydrates: 32 g
- Fiber: 4 g
- Sodium: 563 mg
- Protein: 4 g

Broccoli Egg Muffins

Prep Time: 8-10 min.

Cooking Time: 13-15 min.

Number of Servings: 6

Freestyle Points per Serving: 4

Ingredients:

- 2 cups broccoli, steamed and chopped into small pieces
- Pepper and salt as per taste
- ½ tablespoon Dijon mustard
- 2 green onions, chop into small pieces
- ¾ cup shredded cheddar cheese, reduced fat
- 4 egg whites
- 8 eggs

Directions:

1. Preheat an oven to 350°F.
2. Spray 12 muffins with cooking spray.
3. Take a mixing bowl (either medium or large size), crack and whisk the eggs. Mix in the pepper, salt, mustard, and egg whites.
4. Mix in the cheese, green onions, and broccoli.
5. Add the mix into muffin tins. Bake for 12 minutes or until puffs up.
6. Serve warm.

Nutritional Values (Per Serving):

Calories – 184

Fat – 9g

Saturated Fats – 4g

Trans Fats - 0g

Carbohydrates – 4g

Fiber – 1g

Sodium – 312mg

Protein – 16g

Delicious Almond Pancake

Number of Servings: 6

Prep Time: 10 minutes

Cooking Time: 10 minutes

SmartPoints: 3

Ingredients:

- 6 whole eggs
- ¼ cup almonds, toasted
- 2 ounces cocoa chocolate
- 1/3 cup coconut, shredded
- 1 teaspoon almond extract
- ½ teaspoon baking powder
- ¼ cup of coconut oil
- ¼ cup stevia
- 1 cup almond milk
- Cooking spray as needed
- Pinch of salt

Method:

1. Take a bowl and add coconut flour, stevia, salt, baking powder, coconut and gently stir
2. Add coconut oil, eggs, almond milk, almond extract and stir well
3. Add chocolate, almond and whisk well
4. Take a pan and place it over medium heat, add 2 tablespoons batter, spread into a circle
5. Cook until golden and flip, transfer to pan
6. Repeat with remaining batter
7. Serve and enjoy!

Nutritional Values (Per Serving)

- Calories: 266
- Fat: 13g
- Carbohydrates: 10g
- Protein: 11g

- Saturated Fat: 2g
- Sodium: 242mg
- Fiber: 1g

Homely Chicken Omelet

Number of Servings: 2

Prep Time: 10 minutes

Cooking Time: 10 minutes

SmartPoints: 3

Ingredients:

- 2 bacon slices, cooked and crumbled
- 2 whole eggs
- 1 tablespoon homemade mayonnaise
- 1 tomato, chopped
- 1-ounce rotisserie chicken, shredded
- 1 teaspoon mustard
- 1 small avocado, pitted, peeled and chopped
- Salt and pepper to taste

Method:

1. Take a bowl and add eggs, salt, pepper and whisk well
2. Take a pan and place it over medium heat, add cooking oil, eggs and cook for 5 minutes
3. Add chicken, avocado, tomato, bacon, mayo, and mustard on one half of omelet
4. Fold omelet and cover pan, cook for 5 minutes more
5. Transfer to a serving plate, serve and enjoy!

Nutritional Values (Per Serving)

- Calories: 400
- Fat: 32g
- Carbohydrates: 4g

- Protein: 25g
- Saturated Fat: 7g
- Sodium: 245mg
- Fiber: 1g

Simple Almond Cereal

Number of Servings: 3

Prep Time: 10 minutes

Cooking Time: Nil

SmartPoints: 2

Ingredients:

- 2 tablespoons almond, chopped
- 1/3 cup coconut milk
- 1 tablespoon chia seeds
- 2 tablespoons pepitas, roasted
- Handful of berries
- 1 small banana, chopped
- 1/3 cup water

Method:

1. Take a bowl and add chia seeds, coconut milk, keep it on the side for 5 minutes
2. Take your food processor and add half of pepitas, almonds and pulse them
3. Add this mix to chia seeds
4. Add water and stir
5. Top with remaining pepitas, bananas and blueberries
6. Stir and serve
7. Enjoy!

Nutritional Values (Per Serving)

- Calories: 200
- Fat: 3g
- Carbohydrates: 5g

- Protein: 4g
- Saturated Fat: 1g
- Sodium: 65mg
- Fiber: 1g

Delicious Almond Berry Smoothie

Prep Time: 10 minutes

Cooking Time: Nil

Number of Servings: 2

SmartPoints: 2

Ingredients:

- 1 cup of frozen blueberries
- 1 banana, chopped
- ½ a cup of almond milk
- 1 tablespoon of almond butter
- Water as needed

Method:

1. Add the listed ingredients to the blender and blend them well until you have a smooth texture
2. Add water to thin out the smoothie
3. Chill and enjoy it!

<u>Nutritional Values (Per Serving)</u>

- Calories: 321
- Fat: 11 g
- Saturated Fat: 3 g
- Carbohydrates: 55 g
- Fiber: 4 g
- Sodium: 600 mg
- Protein: 5 g

Simple 3 Ingredient Pancake

Prep Time: 10 minutes

Cooking Time: 10 minutes

Number of Servings: 2

SmartPoints: 2

Ingredients:

- 1 small banana, ripe
- 1 medium egg
- 2 tablespoons wholemeal self-rising flour

Method:

1. Take a medium-sized bowl and add bananas, mash them using a fork
2. Whisk in eggs, flour and mix well to ensure that everything is incorporated well
3. Allow the mixture to sit for 5 minutes
4. Take a nonstick frying pan and grease up the pan with oil
5. Heat the pan over medium heat and spoon 2 tablespoons of your batter
6. Cook each side for 2 minutes until both sides are fully golden
7. Repeat with the remaining batter until they are used up
8. Enjoy!

<u>Nutritional Values (Per Serving)</u>

- Calories: 139
- Fat: 6 g
- Saturated Fat: 0.1 g
- Carbohydrates: 18 g
- Fiber: 3 g
- Sodium: 72 mg
- Protein: 3 g

Chapter 2: Vegetarian And Vegan Recipes

Melon And Watercress Salad

Prep Time: 10 minutes

Cooking Time: Nil

Number of Servings: 4

SmartPoints: 1

Ingredients:

- 3 tablespoons fresh lime juice
- 1 teaspoon date paste
- 1 teaspoon fresh ginger root, minced
- ¼ cup of vegetable oil
- 2 bunches watercress, trimmed and chopped
- 2 and ½ cups watermelon, cubed
- 2 and ½ cups cantaloupe, cubed
- 1/3 cup almonds, sliced

Method:

1. Take a large-sized bowl and add lime juice, ginger, date paste
2. Whisk well and add oil
3. Season with pepper and salt
4. Add watercress, watermelon
5. Toss well
6. Transfer to a serving bowl and garnish with sliced almonds
7. Enjoy!

Nutritional Values (Per Serving)

- Calories: 274
- Fat: 20 g
- Saturated Fat: 6 g
- Carbohydrates: 21 g
- Fiber: 4 g
- Sodium: 420 mg

- Protein: 7 g

Beet And Mushroom Meal

Prep Time: 10 minutes

Cooking Time: 20 minutes

Number of Servings: 4

SmartPoints: 2

Ingredients:

- 4 medium portobello mushroom caps
- ¼ cup lemon juice
- 3 tablespoons olive oil
- 1 small shallot, chopped
- 5 ounces baby kale
- 8 ounces beets, pre-cooked and chopped
- 2 avocados, ripe and thinly sliced

Method:

1. Take a large-sized rimmed baking sheet and spray Portobello mushroom caps with cooking spray
2. Sprinkle ½ a teaspoon of salt
3. Add mushroom to a baking sheet and bake for 20 minutes at 450 degrees Fahrenheit
4. Take a bowl and whisk in lemon juice, olive oil, shallot, ¼ teaspoon of salt, ¼ teaspoon of pepper
5. Add half of the beets and baby kale and toss
6. Divide the mixture amongst serving plates and top with avocado, mushroom
7. Serve with dressing and enjoy!

Nutritional Values (Per Serving)

- Calories: 370
- Fat: 26 g
- Saturated Fat: 4 g
- Carbohydrates: 32 g
- Fiber: 3 g

- Sodium: 393 mg
- Protein: 7 g

Fresh Heirloom Carrot

Prep Time: 10 minutes

Cooking Time: 45 minutes

Number of Servings: 4

SmartPoints: 1

Ingredients:

- 1 bunch heirloom carrots
- 1 tablespoon fresh thyme leaves
- 1 tablespoon date paste
- 1/8 cup fresh orange juice
- 1/8 teaspoon salt

Method:

1. Preheat your oven to 350 degrees Fahrenheit
2. Wash the carrots and discard the green pieces
3. Take a small-sized bowl and add coconut oil, orange juice, salt, and date paste
4. Pour the mixture over carrots and spread on a large-sized baking sheet
5. Sprinkle thyme and roast for 45 minutes
6. Sprinkle salt on top and enjoy!

Nutritional Values (Per Serving)

- Calories: 70
- Fat: 3 g
- Saturated Fat: 1 g
- Carbohydrates: 11 g
- Fiber: 2 g
- Sodium: 186 mg
- Protein: 1 g

Original Avocado Salad

Number of Servings: 3

Prep Time: 10 minutes

Cooking Time: 5 minutes

SmartPoints: 1

Ingredients:

- 1 cup arugula lettuce
- 3 ounces bacon, sliced
- ½ avocado, chopped
- 1 tablespoon lemon juice
- 1 teaspoon olive oil
- 1 tablespoon almonds, chopped
- 1 teaspoon coconut milk

Method:

1. Chop sliced avocado roughly, toss it in a skillet and roast for 5 minutes
2. Once bacon becomes crunchy, add bacon to the salad bowl
3. Add chopped avocado, almonds to the bowl
4. Make seasoning mix by mixing coconut milk, olive oil, and lemon juice
5. Pour dressing over salad and mix well
6. Serve and enjoy!

Nutritional Values (Per Serving)

- Calories: 402
- Fat: 32g
- Carbohydrates: 10g
- Protein: 20g
- Saturated Fat: 8g
- Sodium: 243 mg
- Fiber: 2g

Chapter 3: Chicken And Poultry Recipes

Hearty Balsamic Chicken

Number of Servings: 4

Prep Time: 10 minutes

Cooking Time: 20 minutes

SmartPoints: 3

Ingredients:

- 3 boneless chicken breasts
- Salt and pepper to taste
- ¼ cup all-purpose flour
- 2/3 cup vegetable broth
- 1 and ½ teaspoon of corn starch
- ½ cup raspberry preserve (Sugar-free)
- 1 and ½ tablespoon balsamic vinegar

Method:

1. Cut the chicken into bite-sized portions and season with salt and pepper
2. Dredge the meat into flour and shake off excess
3. Take a nonstick skillet and place it over medium heat
4. Add chicken and cook for 15 minutes, turning once halfway through
5. Remove cooked chicken and transfer to a plate
6. Add cornstarch, chicken broth, raspberry preserve into the skillet and stir in balsamic vinegar (keep the heat on medium)
7. Transfer the cooked chicken to the skillet
8. Cook for 15 minutes more, making sure to turn once
9. Serve and enjoy!

Nutritional Values (Per Serving)

- Calories: 194
- Fat: 15 g
- Saturated Fat: 3 g
- Carbohydrates: 15 g

- Fiber: 3 g
- Sodium: 756 mg
- Protein: 19 g

Epic Mango Chicken

Number of Servings: 4

Prep Time: 10 minutes

Cooking Time: 10 minutes

SmartPoints: 2

Ingredients:

- 2 medium mangoes, peeled and sliced
- 10 ounces of coconut milk
- 4 teaspoons olive oil
- 4 teaspoons curry paste
- 14 ounces chicken breasts, skinless and boneless cut into cubes
- 4 medium shallots
- 1 large English cucumber, seeded and sliced

Method:

1. Slice half of the mangoes and add the halves to a bowl
2. Add mangoes and coconut milk to a blender and blend until you have a smooth puree
3. Keep the mixture on the side
4. Take a large-sized pot and place it over medium heat, add oil and allow the oil to heat up
5. Add curry paste and cook for 1 minute until you have a nice fragrance, add shallots and chicken to the pot and cook for 5 minutes
6. Pour mango puree to the mix and allow it to heat up
7. Serve the cooked chicken with mango puree and cucumbers
8. Enjoy!

Nutritional Values (Per Serving)

- Calories: 400
- Fat: 20 g
- Saturated Fat: 5 g
- Carbohydrates: 31 g
- Fiber: 8 g

- Sodium: 1235 mg
- Protein: 26 g

Thick Broccoli And Cream Soup

Number of Servings: 2

Prep Time: 10 minutes

Cooking Time: 15 minutes

SmartPoints: 2

Ingredients:

- ½ cup heavy cream
- ½ cup of water
- 1 cup broccoli florets
- ¼ cup white onion, chopped
- ¼ teaspoon garlic, diced
- 3 ounces Cheddar cheese, shredded
- 1 ounce's bacon, fried and chopped
- 1 teaspoon butter
- 1 teaspoon dried cilantro
- ¾ teaspoon cayenne pepper

Method:

1. Add water and heavy cream to a saucepan, bring the mix to a boil
2. Add broccoli florets, diced onion, garlic, butter, dried cilantro, cayenne pepper
3. Boil mixture for 10 minutes until broccoli is cooked well
4. Add shredded cheese to boil for 3 minutes more, until cheese melts
5. Once the cheese has melted, blend the soup with help of immersion blender/hand blender
6. Ladle soup into serving bowls and serve
7. Enjoy!

Nutritional Values (Per Serving)

- Calories: 392
- Fat: 33g
- Carbohydrates: 7g

- Protein: 18g
- Saturated Fat: 7g
- Sodium: 698mg
- Fiber: 3g

Roasted Tomato Soup

Number of Servings: 2

Prep Time: 15 minutes

Cooking Time: 15 minutes

SmartPoints: 2

Ingredients:

- 1 cup tomatoes
- 1/3 cup heavy cream
- 1 and ½ cups of water
- 1 tablespoon Italian seasoning
- 1 teaspoon olive oil
- ½ teaspoon chili flakes
- ½ teaspoon salt
- 1 garlic clove, peeled

Method:

1. Make small cuts in tomatoes, add garlic
2. Preheat your oven to 365 degrees F
3. Transfer prepared tomatoes to the baking pan, cook for 10 minutes
4. Transfer baked tomatoes to a food processor, add water, heavy cream, Italian seasoning, olive oil, chili flakes, and salt
5. Process well until smooth
6. Transfer liquid to the saucepan and place it overheat, bring to a boil
7. Lower heat to low and cook for a few minutes, let the soup chill for 5-10 minutes
8. Serve and enjoy once done!

Nutritional Values (Per Serving)

- Calories: 129
- Fat: 12g
- Carbohydrates: 5g
- Protein: 1.3g
- Saturated Fat: 4g
- Sodium: 940mg

- Fiber: 2g

Creative Green Soup

Number of Servings: 3

Prep Time: 10 minutes

Cooking Time: 10-15 minutes

SmartPoints: 3

Ingredients:

- 1 cauliflower head, florets separated
- 1 white onion, chopped
- 1 bay leaf, crushed
- 5 ounces watercress
- 1-quart vegetable stock
- 1 cup of coconut milk
- 7 ounces of spinach leaves
- ¼ cup ghee
- Handful of parsley
- Salt and pepper to taste

Method:

1. Take a pot and place it over medium-high heat, add garlic, onion and stir cook for 4 minutes
2. Add cauliflower, bay leaf and cook for 5 minutes
3. Add watercress, spinach and cook for 3 minutes
4. Add stock, salt, and pepper, bring to a boil
5. Add coconut milk, stir well and use a hand blender to blend well
6. Divide into bowls, serve and enjoy!

Nutritional Values (Per Serving)

- Calories: 230
- Fat: 34g
- Carbohydrates: 5g
- Protein: 7g
- Saturated Fat: 6g

- Sodium: 717mg
- Fiber: 3g

Turkey Green Bean Soup

Prep Time: 8-10 min.

Cooking Time: 25 min.

Number of Servings: 6

Freestyle Points per Serving: 0

Ingredients:

- 1 ½ teaspoon minced garlic
- 1 ½ pound ground turkey breasts, skinless
- 1 cup chopped celery
- ½ cup onion, chopped
- 6 cups chicken broth, fat-free and low-sodium
- ½ cup frozen whole kernel corn
- 1 ½ teaspoon ground cumin
- 1 teaspoon chili powder
- 1 cup carrot, make slices
- ½ cup fresh green beans, make small pieces
- 2 bay leaves
- Cooking oil as needed
- 1 can tomatoes and green chilies, diced and undrained
- 6 tablespoons Monterey Jack cheese, grated
- 1 can kidney beans, rinsed and drained

Directions:

1. Take a skillet or saucepan (medium size preferable); heat it over a medium cooking flame.
2. Add the oil and heat it.
3. Add the celery, onion, garlic, and turkey. Stir and cook for 3 minutes.
4. Add the rest of the ingredient except the cheese.
5. Cover it; boil the mix. Let the mix simmer for about 18-20 minutes.
6. Serve warm with cheese on top.

Nutritional Values (Per Serving):

Calories – 204

Fat – 3g

Saturated Fats – 1g

Trans Fats - 0g

Carbohydrates – 21g

Fiber – 6g

Sodium – 532mg

Protein – 17g

Mesmerizing Orange Baked Chicken

Number of Servings: 4

Prep Time: 10 minutes

Cooking Time: 35 minutes

SmartPoints: 2

Ingredients:

- 2 tablespoons orange juice
- 2 tablespoons Dinon mustard
- ¼ teaspoon salt
- ¾ cup whole wheat crackers, crumbled
- 1 tablespoon orange zest, grated
- 1 shallot, chopped
- ¼ teaspoon black pepper
- 12 ounces chicken thigh, boneless and skinless

Method:

1. Preheat your oven to a temperature of 350 degrees Fahrenheit
2. Take a nonstick baking sheet and spray it with cooking spray
3. Take a small bowl and combine orange juice, salt, and mustard
4. Take a sheet of wax paper and combine cracker crumbs, shallot, orange zest, and pepper

5. Brush up the chicken with the mustard mix and dredge the chicken in the crumbs
6. Firmly place the crumbs to coat all sides of the chicken
7. Place the chicken on your baking sheet
8. Bake for about 15 minutes, making sure to turn it over
9. Bake for another 15 minutes more
10. Serve!

Nutritional Values (Per Serving)

- Calories: 441
- Fat: 12 g
- Saturated Fat: 4 g
- Carbohydrates: 18 g
- Fiber: 3 g
- Sodium: 843 mg
- Protein: 62 g

Cool Sheet-Pan Chicken Asparagus

Number of Servings: 3

Prep Time: 10 minutes

Cooking Time: 25-30 minutes

SmartPoints: 3

Ingredients:

- ½ pounds asparagus, trimmed
- 2 pounds chicken breasts, cut in half to make 4 thin pieces
- 4 sundried tomatoes, cut into strips
- 8 provolone cheese slices
- Salt and pepper to taste

Method:

1. Preheat your oven to 400 degrees F, take a large sheet and grease it well
2. Arrange chicken breasts and asparagus on a sheet pan, top with sundried tomatoes

3. Season well with salt and pepper, transfer to the oven
4. Bake for 25 minutes, remove from oven
5. Top with provolone cheese slices and bake for 3 minutes
6. Dish out, serve, and enjoy!

Nutritional Values (Per Serving)

- Calories: 322
- Fat: 15g
- Carbohydrates: 3g
- Protein: 40g
- Saturated Fat: 3g
- Sodium: 399mg
- Fiber: 1g

Chapter 4: Fish And Seafood Recipes

Awesome Dijon Fish

Prep Time: 5 minutes
Cooking Time: 12 minutes
Number of Servings: 2
SmartPoints: 2

Ingredients:

- 1 perch fillet
- 1 tablespoon Dijon mustard
- 1 and ½ teaspoon lemon juice
- 1 teaspoon Worcestershire sauce
- 2 tablespoons Italian seasoned bread crumbs
- Butter flavored cooking spray as needed

Method:

1. Preheat your oven to 450 degrees Fahrenheit
2. Take an 11 x 7-inch baking dish and arrange your fillets carefully
3. Take a small-sized bowl and add lemon juice, Worcestershire sauce, mustard and mix it well
4. Pour the mix over your fillet
5. Sprinkle a good amount of breadcrumbs
6. Bake for 12 minutes until fish flakes off easily
7. Cut the fillet in half portions and enjoy!

Nutritional Values (Per Serving)

- Calories: 125
- Fat: 2 g
- Saturated Fat: 0.5 g
- Carbohydrates: 6 g
- Fiber: 2 g
- Sodium: 280 mg
- Protein: 21 g

Juicy Shrimp Scampi

Prep Time: 10 minutes

Cooking Time: 5 minutes

Number of Servings: 2

SmartPoints: 2

Ingredients:

- 4 teaspoons olive oil
- 1 and ¼ pound medium shrimp
- 6-8 garlic cloves, minced
- ½ cup low sodium chicken broth
- ½ cup dry white wine
- ¼ cup fresh lemon juice
- 1/3 cup fresh parsley, minced +1 tablespoon extra
- ¼ teaspoon salt
- ¼ teaspoon fresh pepper
- 4 slices lemon

Method:

1. Take a large-sized bowl and place it over medium-high heat
2. Add oil and allow the oil to heat up
3. Add shrimp and cook for 2-3 minutes
4. Add garlic and cook for 30 seconds
5. Take a slotted spoon and carefully transfer the cooked shrimp to your serving platter
6. Add broth, lemon juice, wine, ¼ cup of parsley, salt and pepper to the same skillet and bring the whole mix to a boil
7. Keep boiling until the sauce has been reduced to half
8. Spoon the sauce over the cooked shrimp
9. Garnish with a bit of parsley and lemon
10. Serve and enjoy!

Nutritional Values (Per Serving)

- Calories: 184
- Fat: 3 g
- Saturated Fat: 0.6 g
- Carbohydrates: 6 g
- Fiber: 2 g
- Sodium: 488 mg
- Protein: g

Creamed Halibut

Prep Time: 10 min.

Cooking Time: 15 min.

Number of Servings: 4

SMARTPOINTS PER SERVING: 3

Ingredients:

2 tablespoons butter

¼ cup heavy cream

6 cups fish stock

4 (6 ounce) halibut steak

1 tablespoon each of parsley and thyme

3 tablespoons flour

Salt, ground black pepper and paprika to taste

Directions:

1. In a saucepan or skillet, heat the stock over medium heat setting.
2. Add the halibut and boil the mixture. Allow simmering for about 12 minutes over the low stove flame.
3. Season with ground black pepper and salt to taste. Turn off the heat.
4. Take out the fish and arrange on a serving plate. Also, take out 1 ½ cups of the fish stock.
5. In a saucepan or skillet, heat the butter over medium heat setting.
6. Add the flour and stir well. Add the fish stock and boil the mixture.
7. Add the cream; stir cook for 1 minute. Season with paprika, salt, and pepper.
8. Add the mixture over the prepared steaks. Serve topped with the parsley and thyme.

Nutritional Values (Per Serving):

Calories: 568
Fat: 31g
Saturated Fat: 14g
Trans Fat: 0g

Carbohydrates: 8g
Fiber: 0.5g
Sodium: 814mg
Protein: 47g

Classic Crab Cakes

Prep Time: 10-15 min.

Cooking Time: 30 min.

Number of Servings: 8

SMARTPOINTS PER SERVING: 3

Ingredients:

2 egg whites, beaten

1 whole egg, beaten

16 ounce crab meat

1 cup corn kernels

1 cup crackers, crushed

1/4 cup red bell pepper, minced

4 scallions, chopped fine

2 tablespoons yogurt, fat-free

2 tablespoons mayonnaise

1/4 cup parsley

Juice of 1 lemon

Ground black pepper and salt to taste to taste

Directions:

1. In a mixing bowl (medium-large size), add the scallions, crackers, corn, eggs, black pepper, parsley, lemon juice, mayo, yogurt, ground black pepper, and salt. Combine well.
2. Add the crab meat and combine the mixture. Prepare 8 patties from the mixture and refrigerate for 1 hour.
3. Preheat an oven to 425°F. Grease a baking sheet with some cooking oil.

4. Bake about 25 minutes or until golden brown. Serve warm.

Nutritional Values (Per Serving):

Calories: 103
Fat: 3g
Saturated Fat: 0.5g
Trans Fat: 0g
Carbohydrates: 8g
Fiber: 1g
Sodium: 376mg
Protein: 11.5g

Baked Garlic And Lemon Mahi Mahi

Number of Servings: 3

Prep Time: 10 minutes

Cooking Time: 30 minutes

SmartPoints: 2

Ingredients:

- 1 tablespoon extra-virgin olive oil
- 3 garlic cloves, minced
- 4 pieces (4 ounces each) mahi-mahi fillets
- ½ teaspoon pepper
- Zest from 1 lemon

Method:

1. Take a skillet and place it over medium heat, add oil and let it heat up
2. Add garlic and Sauté until fragrant
3. Add fillets and season with pepper, lemon zest
4. Preheat your oven to 350 degrees F
5. Transfer fish to oven and bake for 30 minutes
6. Serve and enjoy once done!

Nutritional Values (Per Serving)

- Calories: 111
- Fat: 2g
- Carbohydrates: 2g
- Protein: 21g
- Saturated Fat: 1g
- Sodium: 162mg
- Fiber: 0.5g

Lovely Mediterranean Fish

Number of Servings: 4

Prep Time: 10 minutes

Cooking Time: 25 minutes

SmartPoints: 2

Ingredients:

- 2 tablespoons olive oil
- 4 pieces (6 ounces each) fish fillets
- 1 large tomato, chopped
- ¼ cup pitted olives, low sodium
- 2 tablespoons capers
- 1 tablespoon lemon juice
- Salt and pepper to taste

Method:

1. Preheat your oven to 350 degrees F
2. Place olive oil in the middle of a large aluminum foil, put fish in middle and top with tomato, onion, olives, and capers
3. Season well with lemon juice, salt, and pepper
4. Fold in aluminum foil and seal edges well
5. Transfer to baking pan and bake for 25 minutes
6. Serve and enjoy!

Nutritional Values (Per Serving)

- Calories: 210
- Fat: 9g
- Carbohydrates: 7g
- Protein: 27g
- Saturated Fat: 3g
- Sodium: 550mg
- Fiber: 3g

The Pan-Grilled Fish Steaks

Number of Servings: 4

Prep Time: 10 minutes

Cooking Time: 10 minutes

SmartPoints: 2

Ingredients:

- 1 tablespoon olive oil
- 1 garlic clove, minced
- 2 halibut fillets
- 1 teaspoon dried basil
- 1 teaspoon black pepper
- 1 tablespoon lemon juice, freshly squeezed
- 1 tablespoon fresh parsley, chopped

Method:

1. Take a skillet and place it over medium heat, add garlic and Sauté until fragrant
2. Stir in halibut, sear all sides for 2 minutes each
3. Add basil, pepper, lemon juice
4. Cook until juices evaporate, flip the fillet
5. Cook for 5 minutes, garnish with parsley
6. Serve and enjoy!

Nutritional Values (Per Serving)

- Calories: 407
- Fat: 31g
- Carbohydrates: 2g
- Protein: 29g
- Saturated Fat: 9g
- Sodium: 352mg
- Fiber: 0.3g

Classic Mediterranean Fish

Number of Servings: 4

Prep Time: 10 minutes

Cooking Time: 25 minutes

SmartPoints: 2

Ingredients:

- 2 tablespoons olive oil
- 4 pieces (6 ounces each) fish fillets
- 1 large tomato, chopped
- ¼ cup pitted olives, low sodium
- 2 tablespoons capers
- 1 tablespoon lemon juice
- Salt and pepper to taste

Method:

7. Preheat your oven to 350 degrees F
8. Place olive oil in the middle of a large aluminum foil, put fish in middle and top with tomato, onion, olives, and capers
9. Season well with lemon juice, salt, and pepper

10. Fold in aluminum foil and seal edges well
11. Transfer to baking pan and bake for 25 minutes
12. Serve and enjoy!

Nutritional Values (Per Serving)

- Calories: 210
- Fat: 9g
- Carbohydrates: 7g
- Protein: 27g
- Saturated Fat: 3g
- Sodium: 550mg
- Fiber: 3g

Simple Baked Mahi Mahi

Prep Time: 10 minutes

Cooking Time: 30 minutes

Number of Servings: 4

SmartPoints: 2

Ingredients:

- 1 tablespoon extra-virgin olive oil
- 3 garlic cloves, minced
- 4 pieces (4 ounces each) mahi-mahi fillets
- ½ teaspoon pepper
- Zest from 1 lemon

Method:

1. Take a skillet and place it over medium heat, add oil and let it heat up
2. Add garlic and Sauté until fragrant
3. Add fillets and season with pepper, lemon zest
4. Preheat your oven to 350 degrees F
5. Transfer fish to oven and bake for 30 minutes
6. Serve and enjoy once done!

Nutritional Values (Per Serving)

- Calories: 111
- Fat: 2 g
- Saturated Fat: 1 g
- Carbohydrates: 2 g
- Fiber: 0.5 g
- Sodium: 317 mg
- Protein: 21 g

Chapter 5: Beef And Pork Recipes

Caramelized Pork Chops And Onion

Prep Time: 10 minutes

Cooking Time: 30 minutes

Number of Servings: 2

SmartPoints: 3

Ingredients:

- 4 pounds chuck roast
- 4 ounces green chile, chopped
- 2 tablespoons chili powder
- ½ teaspoon dried oregano
- ½ teaspoon ground cumin
- 2 garlic cloves, minced
- Salt as needed

Method:

1. Rub the chops with a seasoning of 1 teaspoon of pepper and 2 teaspoons of salt
2. Take a skillet and place it over medium heat, add oil and allow the oil to heat up
3. Brown the seasoned chop both sides
4. Add water and onion to the skillet and cover, lower down the heat to low and simmer for 20 minutes
5. Turn the chops over and season with more salt and pepper
6. Cover and cook until the water fully evaporates and the beef shows a slightly brown texture
7. Remove the chops and serve with a topping of the caramelized onion
8. Serve and enjoy!

<u>**Nutritional Values (Per Serving)**</u>

- Calories: 47
- Fat: 4 g
- Saturated Fat: 1 g
- Carbohydrates: 4 g

- Fiber: 1 g
- Sodium: 240 mg
- Protein: 0.5g

Mustard Lamb Cutlets

Prep Time: 10 minutes

Cooking Time: 10 minutes

Number of Servings: 2

SmartPoints: 3

Ingredients:

- 1 tablespoon Dijon mustard
- 1 tablespoon honey
- 2 tablespoons white wine vinegar
- 15 ounces lamb cutlet, trimmed
- 1 and ½ cup brown rice, cooked
- 2 cups baby spinach leaves, shredded

Method:

1. Take a small-sized bowl and add mustard, honey, vinegar and mix well
2. Preheat your BBQ grill to high
3. Cook the cutlets for about 2 minutes per side to ensure that they are cooked well
4. Brush half of your mustard mix near the end of the cooking
5. Take a microwave-safe bowl and add the rice, place them in your microwave and cook
6. Stir in spinach leaves while the rice is hot
7. Divide the rice amongst your serving plates and top up with the grille cutlets
8. Drizzle the remaining mustard mix on top and enjoy!

Nutritional Values (Per Serving)

- Calories: 1507
- Fat: 124 g
- Saturated Fat: 26 g
- Carbohydrates: 55 g
- Fiber: 10 g
- Sodium: 370 mg
- Protein: 54 g

Beef Broccoli Dinner

Prep Time: 8-10 min.

Cooking Time: 10-15 min.

Number of Servings: 4

Freestyle Points per Serving: 3

Ingredients:

- 3/4 pound lean sirloin beef
- 1/4 teaspoon salt
- 5 cups broccoli florets
- 1 cup chicken broth, reduced-sodium
- 2 ½ tablespoon cornstarch
- 2 teaspoon canola oil
- 1/4 cup water
- 1/4 teaspoon red pepper flakes
- 2 tablespoon minced garlic
- 1/4 cup soy sauce
- 1 tablespoon minced ginger root

Directions:

1. Combine the 2 tablespoons cornstarch and salt; coat the beef with it.
2. Take a skillet or saucepan (medium size preferable); heat it over a medium cooking flame.
3. Add the oil and heat it.
4. Add the beef and cook, while stirring, until turns evenly brown for 3-4 minutes. Set the beef aside.
5. Add ½ cup of the broth, broccoli and cook for 2-3 minutes.
6. Add the garlic, ginger, and pepper flakes. Simmer the mix for 1 more minute.
7. Take a mixing bowl (either medium or large size), add in the rest of the broth, soy sauce, and rest of the cornstarch in the bowl to mix well with each other.
8. Turn down heat; cover and simmer for 1 minute. Mix in the broth mix and beef; serve warm.

Nutritional Values (Per Serving):

Calories – 253

Fat – 11g

Saturated Fats – 3g

Trans Fats - 0g

Carbohydrates – 7g

Fiber – 1g

Sodium – 753mg

Protein – 27g

Roast Taco Wraps

Prep Time: 8-10 min.

Cooking Time: 0 min.

Number of Servings: 7

Freestyle Points per Serving: 6

Ingredients:

- ½ pound cooked roast beef, make slices
- 2 make slices tomatoes
- ¼ teaspoon pepper
- 7 pieces tortilla
- 2 teaspoon Dijon mustard
- 1/3 cup basil
- 1/3 cup mayo
- 2 cup shredded lettuce
- ¼ teaspoon salt

Directions:

1. Take a mixing bowl (either medium or large size), add in the pepper, mustard, salt, basil, and mayo in the bowl to mix well with each other.
2. Arrange the tortillas and spread the mix; top with some lettuce, roast beef, and tomatoes. Roll the tortillas and serve.

Nutritional Values (Per Serving):

Calories – 193

Fat – 9g

Saturated Fats – 2g

Trans Fats - 0g

Carbohydrates – 16g

Fiber – 1g

Sodium – 647mg

Protein – 12g

Grilled Spiced Chops

Prep Time: 8-10 min.

Cooking Time: 8 min.

Number of Servings: 4

Freestyle Points per Serving: 6

Ingredients:

- 2 teaspoons brown sugar
- 1 1/3 pound boneless pork chops
- 2 teaspoons vegetable oil
- 2 teaspoons sweet paprika
- 1/2 teaspoon ground garlic powder
- 1/2 teaspoon ground cinnamon
- 1/2 teaspoon kosher salt
- 1/2 teaspoon ground ginger

Directions:

1. Take a mixing bowl (either medium or large size), add in the paprika, sugar, chili powder, cinnamon, salt, ginger, and garlic powder in the bowl to mix well with each other.
2. Rub over the chops.
3. Preheat your grill over medium-high temperature setting.
4. Grill 3-4 minutes for each side; until cooks well.
5. Serve warm.

Nutritional Values (Per Serving):

Calories – 367

Fat – 23g

Saturated Fats – 3g

Trans Fats - 0g

Carbohydrates – 3g

Fiber – 0g

Sodium – 283mg

Protein – 36g

Beef Stuffed Zucchini

Prep Time: 10 min.
Cooking Time: 25-30 min.
Number of Servings: 8
SMARTPOINTS PER SERVING: 7

Ingredients:

½ cup mozzarella cheese

½ cup cheddar cheese

4 medium zucchini, split lengthwise

10 ounce beef

2 medium tomatoes, peeled and pureed

Ground black pepper and salt to taste

1 clove garlic, minced

1 small onion, diced

Directions:

1. Preheat an oven to 400°F. Grease a baking pan with some cooking oil.
2. Hollow out the zucchini halves and set aside. Chop the zucchini hollowed out the flesh and set aside.
3. In a saucepan or skillet, heat the oil over medium heat setting.

4. Sauté the onions until it becomes softened and translucent. Add the garlic and cook for 1 minute.
5. Add the ground beef and stir well. Season with ground black pepper and salt to taste.
6. Add the pureed tomatoes and zucchini flesh; stir cook for 6-7 minutes. Add half portion cheese and cook until it melts completely.
7. Stuff the mixture in the zucchini halves. Arrange over prepared baking dish and top with the remaining cheeses.
8. Bake for 15 minutes or until the cheese melts. Serve warm.

Nutritional Values (Per Serving):

Calories: 179
Fat: 13g
Saturated Fat: 5g
Trans Fat: 0g
Carbohydrates: 9g
Fiber: 2g
Sodium: 473mg
Protein: 9g

Subtle Herbed Beef Roast

Number of Servings: 3

Prep Time: 10 minutes

Cooking Time: 60-70 minutes

SmartPoints: 3

Ingredients:

- 1-pound rump roast, boneless
- 1 tablespoon yellow mustard
- 1 teaspoon dried thyme
- ½ teaspoon dried rosemary
- 1 teaspoon dried parsley flakes
- Salt and pepper to taste
- ½ cup beef bone broth

- 4 garlic cloves, peeled and halved
- 2 yellow onions, quartered

Method:

1. Pat your roast dry with a towel, rub roast with mustard spices all over
2. Place rump roast in roasting pan, pour beef broth
3. Scatter garlic and onions around meat, transfer to a preheated oven (360 degrees F)
4. Roast for 30 minutes, lower heat to 220 degrees F, roast for 30-40 minutes more
5. Serve and enjoy!

Nutritional Values (Per Serving)

- Calories: 316
- Fat: 13g
- Carbohydrates: 2g
- Protein: 47g
- Saturated Fat: 4g
- Sodium: 494 mg
- Fiber: 0.5g

Purely Spanish Pork Cutlets And Onion

Prep Time: 10 minutes

Cooking Time: 10 minutes

Number of Servings: 4

SmartPoints: 4

Ingredients:

- 1 tablespoon olive oil
- 2 pork cutlets
- 1 bell pepper, deveined and sliced
- 1 Spanish onion, chopped
- 2 garlic cloves, minced
- ½ teaspoon hot sauce
- ½ teaspoon mustard
- ½ teaspoon paprika
- Salt and pepper to taste

Method:

1. Take a large saucepan, add olive oil and place it over medium-high heat
2. Let it heat up, add pork cutlets and fry for 3-4 minutes until golden and crispy on both sides
3. Lower temperature to medium and add bell pepper, Spanish onion, garlic, hot sauce, mustard and cook for 3 minutes until veggies are tender
4. Sprinkle paprika, salt, pepper and serve
5. Enjoy!

Nutritional Values (Per Serving)

- Calories: 24
- Fat: 3 g
- Saturated Fat: 1 g
- Carbohydrates: 2 g
- Fiber: 0.8 g
- Sodium: 219 mg

- Protein: 40 g

Chapter 6: Dessert

Fine Baked Apple

Prep Time: 5 minutes

Cooking Time: 20 minutes

Number of Servings: 2

SmartPoints: 0

Ingredients:

- 1 Fuji Apple
- Raisins as needed
- Cinnamon as needed

Method:

1. Preheat your oven to 347 degrees Fahrenheit
2. Core the apples
3. Stuff them with cinnamon and raisins
4. Transfer to the oven and bake for 20 minutes
5. Serve and enjoy!

Nutritional Values (Per Serving)

- Calories: 95
- Fat: 0.2 g
- Saturated Fat: 0.1 g
- Carbohydrates: 42 g
- Fiber: 5 g
- Sodium: 30 mg
- Protein: 0.43 g

Healthy Bean Balls

Prep Time: 10 minutes

Cooking Time: Nil

Number of Servings: 2

SmartPoints: 2

Ingredients:

- ½ cup dates
- ½ cup dried berries and cherries
- ½ cup almonds, ground
- 2 tablespoons cocoa
- 3 and ¾ cups black beans
- 1 small orange, zest
- Cocoa, coconut, toasted pistachios as a topping

Method:

1. Take a food processor and add dates, ground almond, cocoa, cherries, black bean, and orange zest
2. Process well until finely chopped up
3. Use your hand to make balls out of the mixture into balls
4. Garnish the balls with toasted cocoa, coconut, and pistachios
5. Serve and enjoy!

Nutritional Values (Per Serving)

- Calories: 366
- Fat: 14 g
- Saturated Fat: 3 g
- Carbohydrates: 99 g
- Fiber: 10 g
- Sodium: 129 mg
- Protein: 8 g

Cool Carrot Balls

Prep Time: 10 minutes

Cooking Time: Nil

Number of Servings: 4

SmartPoints: 2

Ingredients:

- 6 Medjool dates pitted
- 1 carrot, grated
- ¼ cup raw walnuts
- ¼ cup unsweetened coconut, shredded
- 1 teaspoon nutmeg
- 1/8 teaspoon salt

Method:

1. Take a food processor and add dates, ¼ cup of grated carrots, salt coconut, nutmeg
2. Mix well and puree the mixture
3. Add the walnuts and remaining ¼ cup of carrots
4. Pulse the mixture until you have a clunky texture
5. Form balls using your hand and roll them up in coconut
6. Top with carrots and chill
7. Enjoy!

Nutritional Values (Per Serving)

- Calories: 326
- Fat: 16 g
- Saturated Fat: 4 g
- Carbohydrates: 42 g
- Fiber: 4 g
- Sodium: 203 mg
- Protein: 3 g

Applesauce Bean Brownies

Prep Time: 8-10 min.

Cooking Time: 30-35 min.

Number of Servings: 12

Freestyle Points per Serving: 1

Ingredients:

- ¼ cup all-purpose flour
- 1/3 cup unsweetened cocoa powder
- ½ teaspoon baking powder
- ½ teaspoon salt
- ¼ cup applesauce, unsweetened
- 1 ½ cups black beans
- ¼ cup blackstrap molasses

Directions:

1. Lightly grease a baking dish (8x8) with cooking spray. Preheat an oven to 375°F.
2. Puree the beans in the blender and pour in a mixing bowl.
3. Ad and mix in the baking powder, salt, applesauce, and molasses.
4. Stir in the flour and cocoa powder; mix well.
5. Add the batter in prepared dish; bake until cooked through for about 35 minutes.

Nutritional Values (Per Serving):

Calories – 143

Fat – 1g

Saturated Fats – 0g

Trans Fats - 0g

Carbohydrates – 32g

Fiber – 3g

Sodium – 263mg

Protein – 3g

Pumpkin Cake Muffins

Prep Time: 8-10 min.

Cooking Time: 20-22 min.

Number of Servings: 24

Freestyle Points per Serving: 2

Ingredients:

- 2 cups pumpkin puree
- 1 cup water
- 1 box yellow cake mix, sugar-free

Directions:

1. Take 24 muffin tins and line them with liner. Preheat an oven to 350°F.
2. Take a mixing bowl (either medium or large size), add and mix all the ingredients in the bowl to mix well with each other.
3. Add into the muffin tins; bake for 22 minutes or until tops are lightly browned.

Nutritional Values (Per Serving):

Calories – 89

Fat – 2g

Saturated Fats – 1g

Trans Fats - 0g

Carbohydrates – 17g

Fiber – 1g

Sodium – 126mg

Protein – 2g

Fried Up Sliced Apples

Prep Time: 10 minutes

Cooking Time: 10 minutes

Number of Servings: 4

SmartPoints: 1

Ingredients:

- ½ cup of coconut oil
- ¼ cup date paste
- 2 tablespoons ground cinnamon
- 4 Granny Smith apples, peeled, cored and sliced

Method:

1. Take a large-sized skillet and place it over medium heat
2. Add oil and allow the oil to heat up
3. Stir in cinnamon and date paste into the oil
4. Add cut up apples and cook for 5:8 minutes until crispy
5. Enjoy!

Nutritional Values (Per Serving)

- Calories: 368
- Fat: 23 g
- Saturated Fat: 10 g
- Carbohydrates: 44 g
- Fiber: 12 g
- Sodium: 182 mg
- Protein: 1 g

Fluffy Almond Pancakes

Number of Servings: 6

Prep Time: 10 minutes

Cooking Time: 10 minutes

SmartPoints: 3

Ingredients:

- 6 whole eggs
- ¼ cup almonds, toasted
- 2 ounces cocoa chocolate
- 1/3 cup coconut, shredded
- 1 teaspoon almond extract
- ½ teaspoon baking powder
- ¼ cup of coconut oil
- ¼ cup stevia
- 1 cup almond milk
- Cooking spray as needed
- Pinch of salt

Method:

8. Take a bowl and add coconut flour, stevia, salt, baking powder, coconut and gently stir
9. Add coconut oil, eggs, almond milk, almond extract and stir well
10. Add chocolate, almond and whisk well
11. Take a pan and place it over medium heat, add 2 tablespoons batter, spread into a circle
12. Cook until golden and flip, transfer to pan
13. Repeat with remaining batter
14. Serve and enjoy!

Nutritional Values (Per Serving)

- Calories: 266
- Fat: 13g
- Carbohydrates: 10 g
- Protein: 11 g
- Saturated Fat: 2 g
- Sodium: 124 mg
- Fiber: 1g

Printed in the USA
CPSIA information can be obtained
at www.ICGtesting.com
LVHW080107110224
771523LV00005B/755